HAND SURGERY RECOVERY DIET

Nourishing Recovery And Understanding Dietary Solutions For Chronic Pain Relief And Bone Healing

DR LUCAS KAYCE

© [Dr Lucas Kayce] [2024]. All rights reserved.

Except for brief quotations included in critical reviews and certain other noncommercial uses allowed by copyright law, no part of this book may be reproduced, distributed, or transmitted in any form or by any means, including photocopying, recording, or other electronic or mechanical methods, without the publisher's prior written permission.

DISCLAIMER

This book about illness and nutrition is not meant to replace expert medical advice, diagnosis, or treatment; rather, it is meant purely for informational reasons. This book's content is founded on broad concepts and recommendations for managing diseases and nutrition.

Before adopting any major dietary or lifestyle changes, readers are recommended to speak with a qualified healthcare provider, such as a licensed physician or registered dietitian, especially if they have pre-existing medical concerns. Everybody has different health demands, so what works for one person might not work for another.

The use of the information provided in this book may have unfavorable repercussions or consequences, for which the author and publisher disclaim all liability. No disease is meant to be identified, treated, cured, or prevented by the information provided.

The book may include contain references to medical literature or research findings; however readers are urged to independently confirm this material and contact reliable sources.

It is important to remember that the fields of nutrition and medicine are always changing, and that new findings could have an impact on the advice offered in this book. As a result, readers are urged to keep up with the most recent advancements in healthcare and, when in doubt, seek professional counsel.

By reading this book, readers agree that they are in charge of their own health decisions and release the author and publisher from any liability arising from the use of the material in the book, whether direct or indirect.

TABLE OF CONTENTS

ABOUT THE BOOK

The book "Hand Surgery Recovery Diet" is a priceless tool that discusses the importance of nutrition in the healing process after hand surgery. Understanding the value of a holistic approach to healing, the book starts with a summary of hand surgery, stressing the complex relationship between nutritional requirements and surgical procedures.

The reader learns about preoperative nutrition standards, talking to surgeons, and mentally preparing for hand surgery. The book then moves smoothly into the critical early postoperative days, providing helpful advice on managing pain, adjusting to postoperative dietary restrictions, and immediate postoperative care. The fundamental knowledge in this section prepares the reader for the main focus of the book, Nutritional Essentials for Recovery.

Here, the book dives into the finer points of nutrition, emphasizing the value of foods high in protein for tissue regeneration, the function that vitamins and minerals play in healing, and the necessity of maintaining adequate hydration. It goes beyond standard nutritional guidance by offering modified eating techniques, like foods that are simple to consume, advice on how to prepare meals, and portion control that is specifically designed to support recovery.

The book also discusses the connection between diet and reducing inflammation, outlining an anti-inflammatory diet and instructing readers on how to include foods high in omega-3 fatty acids and other naturally occurring anti-inflammatory components.

The need to eat a balanced diet is then emphasized, along with tips for including whole grains for long-lasting energy, dairy, and calcium to support bone health.

Setting itself apart from other materials, the book discusses possible interactions between medication and nutrition, providing advice on how to modify one's diet for the best possible pain management. As the book moves into the recovery stage, it highlights the value of exercise and provides nutritional support techniques, such as increasing muscle and flexibility.

Recognizing that healing is a holistic process, the book discusses mental health during the healing phase. Readers will gain important knowledge on stress management strategies, problem-solving strategies, and the critical role that diet plays in maintaining mental health. The last few chapters walk people through the process of gradually returning to a regular diet, focusing on long-term dietary guidelines, a gradual reintroduction of foods, and progress monitoring with medical professionals.

"Hand Surgery Recovery Diet" is essentially a comprehensive guide that offers evidence-based, doable techniques to maximize the healing process in addition to acknowledging the complex relationship between nutrition and hand surgery recovery. This book is an essential resource for anyone managing their recuperation after hand surgery, whether they are medical experts or just folks trying to get well.

CHAPTER ONE

HAND SURGERY RECOVERY DIET OVERVIEW

COMPREHENDING THE RECUPERATION AFTER HAND SURGERY

For those who have surgery to treat a range of hand-related ailments and injuries, hand surgery recovery is an essential stage of the rehabilitation process. To restore optimal function and relieve discomfort, this complex area of medicine focuses on the diagnosis and treatment of conditions affecting the hand, wrist, and forearm. After hand surgery, the healing phase is critical to favorable results. It includes a multifaceted strategy that includes appropriate post-operative care, rehabilitation activities, and sufficient nutrition in the healing process.

A SYNOPSIS OF HAND SURGERY

A summary of hand surgery's many uses shows that it can be used to cure anything from traumas and congenital abnormalities to long-term ailments like arthritis. To improve hand functionality, surgeons may undertake procedures including nerve decompressions, joint replacements, tendon repairs, or corrective surgeries. The nature of the surgery and its intricacy can have a big impact on how long the recovery period takes and what needs to be done throughout it. To maximize the benefits of the surgical procedure, patients must follow the recommended rehabilitation procedures throughout this phase.

THE ROLE OF NUTRITION IN HEALING

Following hand surgery, nutrition is crucial to the healing process since it affects the body's capacity to repair, regenerate tissues, and regain strength. It is impossible to exaggerate the role that nutrition plays in healing because the body needs certain vitamins, minerals, and other vital nutrients to promote healing and reduce difficulties.

Sufficient consumption of protein is especially important since it facilitates the creation of new tissues and encourages general tissue healing. Furthermore, nutrients like zinc and vitamins like C are essential for the synthesis of collagen, which maintains the integrity of the hand's connective tissues.

Incorporating a nutrient-dense, well-balanced diet is crucial for boosting immunity, lowering inflammation, and promoting the body's natural healing process. Eating a healthy diet not only speeds up the healing process but also lowers the chance of surgical complications like infections.

It is frequently recommended that patients collaborate closely with healthcare providers, such as nutritionists, to create individualized eating regimens that meet their unique requirements and promote the best possible outcomes for their recuperation.

Comprehending the recuperation from hand surgery entails realizing the complexity of hand surgeries, valuing the many surgical techniques, and realizing the critical role that diet plays in the healing process.

When it comes to promoting the restoration of optimal hand function for patients undergoing hand surgery and guaranteeing excellent hand surgery results, the cooperation of surgical experience, rehabilitative care, and nutritional assistance is essential.

CHAPTER TWO

GETTING READY FOR HAND SURGERY

SURGEON CONSULTATION

One of the most important steps in getting ready for hand surgery is to see a surgeon. It gives the patient a chance to go through any worries they may have, ask any questions they may have, and get a thorough explanation of the surgery that is going to take place. In the consultation, the hand surgeon will review the possible risks and benefits of surgery, as well as review the patient's medical history and determine the severity of the hand disease. The patient should also reveal any allergies, drugs, or underlying medical conditions that could affect their recovery from surgery at this time.

In addition, the surgeon will go over the specifics of the surgery, including expected results and possible side effects. This enables the patient to choose their course of treatment with knowledge. The consultation helps allay any fears the patient may have over the impending surgery and is an open discussion that strengthens the doctor-patient bond.

GUIDELINES FOR PREOPERATIVE NUTRITION

An essential component of any surgical operation, including hand surgery, is a healthy diet. Following certain dietary recommendations during the preoperative phase can improve the body's capacity for effective healing and recovery.

Consuming enough protein is vital because it promotes tissue healing and aids in the synthesis of collagen, which is a key component of skin and connective tissues.

A well-rounded diet high in vitamins and minerals, especially zinc and vitamin C, can help promote a more favorable healing process. These nutrients support wound healing and immune system performance. Patients may be encouraged to cut back on processed meals and sugars while increasing their intake of fruits, vegetables, and lean meats.

Maintaining proper hydration is crucial since dehydration can obstruct the healing process. Patients should make an effort to keep their fluid levels in check by drinking water and limiting their intake of sugary or caffeinated drinks. By adhering to these preoperative dietary recommendations, you can enhance your body's preparedness for surgery and facilitate a quicker recovery.

MENTAL SURGERY PREPARATION

A patient's psychological state has a major influence on the entire surgical experience and recovery, therefore mental preparation is an essential part of the preoperative process. Mental well-being requires acknowledging and treating any worry or fear related to the procedure. It is encouraged for patients to communicate honestly with their healthcare staff about their expectations and concerns.

Preoperative stress can be effectively managed by using relaxation methods like deep breathing exercises or meditation.

Creating a network of support, consisting of loved ones, close friends, or a mental health expert, can offer emotional support throughout this trying period. Having a clear understanding of the surgical procedure, anticipated results, and probable obstacles can boost confidence and lessen anxiety.

Furthermore, patients can gain from having reasonable expectations regarding the length of their rehabilitation and the rate at which their hand function will gradually improve. Being mentally ready for surgery not only makes the procedure go more smoothly but also improves the quality of life in general while recovering.

CHAPTER THREE

THE INITIAL DAYS FOLLOWING SURGERY

QUICK POSTOPERATIVE TREATMENT

The immediate postoperative care following surgery is essential to the patient's health and recuperation. To guarantee stability, the medical staff keeps a careful eye on vital signs like blood pressure, oxygen saturation, and heart rate. Usually, the patient is sent to a recovery room where they receive specialized care and are closely monitored by medical experts with training. During this stage, it is crucial to keep an eye out for any indications of problems or anesthesia-related side effects.

PAIN CONTROL

To improve patient comfort and speed up the healing process, pain management is a crucial component of postoperative treatment. Several approaches can be used, including the use of regional anesthetic procedures or the injection of analgesic drugs. The type of surgery, the patient's past medical history, and their unique pain threshold all influence the choice of pain management technique. Assessments are carried out regularly to evaluate the efficacy of pain management strategies and modify the treatment plan as necessary.

FIRST NUTRITIONAL LIMITATIONS

In the initial postoperative days following surgery, initial dietary restrictions are frequently instituted to facilitate the healing process and avert problems. Certain food types can be difficult for the body to handle, and there may be a temporary compromise to the digestive system.

A more regular diet may be gradually offered after the introduction of clear liquids, depending on the patient's tolerance and the specifics of the surgical treatment. Foods high in nutrients are frequently given priority to aid in the body's healing and strengthen the immune system.

TIPS FOR HYDRATION

Maintaining general health and facilitating the body's removal of drugs and anesthetics require adequate hydration throughout the postoperative phase. To guarantee adequate hydration following surgery, intravenous fluids are frequently given, particularly if the patient is unable to swallow drinks.

The patient must adhere to any recommended hydration regimen, which may involve consuming both water and electrolyte-rich liquids. Sufficient water promotes the body's natural healing processes and helps avoid issues like dehydration.

Careful attention to immediate postoperative care, efficient pain management, adherence to initial dietary restrictions, and a priority for adequate hydration are all necessary during the first few days following surgery. Together, these elements facilitate a more seamless recuperation process, reducing risks and enhancing the patient's general health.

To facilitate a smooth transition for patients from the surgical operation to the ensuing phases of rehabilitation, healthcare professionals are essential in helping patients through this crucial period.

CHAPTER FOUR

MODIFIED CONSUMPTION PATTERNS

EASY-TO-EAT MEALS

Those who struggle with chewing, swallowing, or other dietary restrictions should prioritize easy-to-eat meals while implementing an adapted eating approach. These foods usually have a soft texture, are readily absorbed, and require little chewing effort. Easy-to-eat options include pureed fruits and vegetables, smoothies, yogurt, and well-cooked grains. By including certain foods in the diet, you may make sure that people who have particular eating disorders get the nutrients they need without overtaxing their digestive systems.

MEAL PREPARATION ADVICE

A well-thought-out meal plan is essential to a modified eating approach, which tries to make things easier for those with a range of medical conditions. Focusing on cooking techniques like steaming, boiling, or slow cooking that improve the softness and palatability of food is one important strategy. Furthermore, preparing purees or finely chopped meals in blenders or food processors can help individuals who struggle with swallowing or chewing. Nutrient-dense foods should always come first because this will guarantee that meals stay balanced even if their texture changes.

Meal planning and frequency should also be taken into consideration. For people with particular medical issues, dividing meals into smaller, more frequent amounts can help with overall digestion and minimize mealtime tiredness. Furthermore, it might improve the person's involvement and contentment with the modified eating plan to include them in meal preparation whenever feasible.

PORTION MANAGEMENT FOR HEALING

For those who are on a healing journey in particular, portion management is an essential component of an adjusted eating plan. Limiting portion sizes guarantees that the body gets the nutrients it needs without taxing the digestive system or adding too many calories.

Meals that are smaller and more balanced might make eating more comfortable, especially for those who are recuperating from surgery, sickness, or long-term medical conditions.

It is imperative to customize portion sizes to meet the demands of each individual, accounting for variables like age, weight, and certain medical problems. To find the right portion sizes that support each person's recovery objectives, it is essential to speak with medical specialists or nutritionists. Nutrient-dense snacks can also be spread out throughout the day to promote the healing process without piling too much strain on the digestive system in addition to meals. All things considered, the effectiveness of an adjusted eating plan intended to support healing and general well-being depends heavily on a careful approach to portion control.

CHAPTER FIVE

FOODS THAT HELP REDUCE INFLAMMATION

BASICS OF AN ANTI-INFLAMMATORY DIET

The cornerstone of controlling inflammation in the body, which is essential for both preventing and treating several medical disorders, is an anti-inflammatory diet. This dietary approach's main objective is to lessen chronic inflammation, which is linked to several illnesses, such as autoimmune disorders, arthritis, and cardiovascular problems. One of the main goals of an anti-inflammatory diet is to minimize the intake of refined and processed meals and to encourage the consumption of complete, nutrient-dense foods.

An anti-inflammatory diet's mainstay is a range of vibrant fruits and vegetables, which are high in phytochemicals and antioxidants. These substances aid in the decrease of inflammation by scavenging free radicals and oxidative stress.

Additionally, important ingredients are whole grains, legumes, nuts, and seeds, which offer vital minerals and fiber that promote general health. Conversely, processed foods, high levels of saturated fats, and refined sugars are prohibited since they exacerbate inflammation and counteract the anti-inflammatory effect.

ADDITION OF OMEGA-3 FATTY ACIDS

Omega-3 fatty acids are essential for reducing inflammation and enhancing general health. The anti-inflammatory qualities of these vital fats—which are mostly present in fatty fish like salmon, mackerel, and sardines—as well as flaxseeds, chia seeds, and walnuts, have been the subject of much research. The body produces inflammatory mediators differently when exposed to the two primary forms of omega-3 fatty acids, eicosapentaenoic acid (EPA) and docosahexaenoic acid (DHA). This is how these fatty acids reduce inflammation.

Apart from their immediate anti-inflammatory properties, omega-3 fatty acids also support the preservation of cellular membrane pliability and integrity, which impacts the inflammatory response differently. People who want to lower inflammation levels should routinely include these omega-3 sources in their diet.

Under the advice of a healthcare provider, omega-3 supplements, such as fish oil capsules or algae-based substitutes for vegetarians or vegans, may be taken into consideration in situations when dietary intake may be inadequate.

FOODS THAT NATURALLY REDUCE INFLAMMATION

Many foods are known to have inherent anti-inflammatory qualities, providing a wide variety of choices for people looking to control inflammation with their diet. For example, curcumin, a substance with strong anti-inflammatory and antioxidant properties, is found in turmeric. Adding turmeric to soups, smoothies, or curries is a tasty way to reap its health benefits.

Another spice that has strong anti-inflammatory qualities is ginger. Ginger has long been prized for its capacity to lessen pain and inflammation, whether it is added to drinks, stir-fries, or other meals. Antioxidants and flavonoids, which are abundant in berries, especially blueberries, contribute to their anti-inflammatory properties. These colorful fruits can be a tasty method to help inflammation reduction when added to salads, breakfast bowls, or snacks.

The anti-inflammatory diet plan entails giving preference to complete, high-nutrient meals, reducing processed and refined foods, including omega-3 fatty acids from various sources, and including foods that naturally have anti-inflammatory qualities. People can promote long-term health and well-being by adopting a balanced and inflammation-resistant lifestyle through thoughtful daily food choices.

CHAPTER SIX

KEEPING YOUR DIET BALANCED

INCLUDING VEGETABLES AND FRUITS

A balanced diet, which includes a range of nutrients to support various body processes, is essential for general health and well-being. Including a wide variety of fruits and vegetables in your diet is essential to a balanced diet. These vibrant, nutrient-dense foods include vital vitamins, minerals, fiber, and antioxidants. A wide range of nutrients is ensured when you eat a rainbow of fruits and vegetables, which promotes optimal health and lowers the risk of chronic diseases.

ENTIRE GRAINS FOR LONG-TERM ENERGY

A key component of maintaining energy levels throughout the day is whole grains. Whole grains, as opposed to refined grains, are a great source of fiber, vitamins, minerals, and complex carbohydrates since they contain the bran, germ, and endosperm. Foods like quinoa, brown rice, oats, and whole wheat help to deliver energy gradually, reducing blood sugar spikes and crashes. Whole grains provide long-lasting energy that enhances mental clarity, physical stamina, and weight management by encouraging fullness.

CALCIUM AND DAIRY FOR HEALTHY BONES

One of the most important sources of calcium, which is necessary for strong and healthy bones, is dairy products. Including dairy products in your diet—whether it be cheese, yogurt, or milk—helps you fulfill your daily calcium needs, maintaining bone density and warding off diseases like osteoporosis. Almond or soy milk are two examples of fortified plant-based milk substitutes that can be great sources of calcium for people who are lactose intolerant or prefer non-dairy options. Incorporating additional calcium-rich foods like tofu, fortified orange juice, and leafy green vegetables can also improve bone health in general.

Making sure you are getting enough dairy or calcium-rich substitutes is especially important for growing people (like children and adolescents) and people who are more likely to experience problems with their bones (such as postmenopausal women). The interplay of calcium, vitamin D, and other nutrients present in dairy products is crucial for calcium absorption and use, underscoring the significance of a well-balanced diet in fostering ideal bone health.

Eating a balanced diet means including a variety of food groups that together supply the nutrients required for good health. An array of vibrant fruits and vegetables, whole grains for long-lasting energy, and sufficient dairy or calcium-rich substitutes are all components of a well-balanced diet that promotes longevity, mental clarity, and physical health.

CHAPTER SEVEN

MEDICATION AND DIETARY CONSIDERATIONS

INTERACTIONS BETWEEN DRUGS

The effectiveness and safety of pharmaceutical therapies are significantly influenced by drug interactions. Interactions between medication and nutrition are intricate and multidimensional. The absorption, metabolism, and efficacy of medication can be affected by specific foods and nutrients. To guarantee the best possible treatment outcomes, patients and healthcare practitioners must understand these connections.

How particular meals may impact the absorption of medications is a crucial component of dietary concerns in medicine. While certain medications absorb best when taken empty-handed, others could absorb better when taken with food. For example, some medicines work better when on an empty stomach since food can decrease the amount of the antibiotic that is absorbed. However, to reduce gastrointestinal adverse effects, some medications—especially those for illnesses like osteoporosis or arthritis—may be taken with meals.

Furthermore, the body's metabolism of several nutrients and drugs may be affected by their interactions. One well-known item that can obstruct the liver's ability to properly metabolize a variety of drugs is grapefruit juice. Due to this interaction, the drug may be more concentrated in the blood, which could have harmful or toxic effects. Healthcare professionals must be aware of these interactions when prescribing drugs and patients must follow dietary recommendations for the best possible drug efficacy.

MODIFYING NUTRITION TO MANAGE PAIN

Another important factor to take into account when managing pain is food, particularly for those with chronic pain disorders. In addition to having a big impact on inflammation, nutrition can either exacerbate or lessen pain symptoms.

Consuming a diet high in anti-inflammatory foods, like fruits, vegetables, and omega-3 fatty acids, may help lessen pain and inflammation brought on by illnesses like arthritis.

On the other hand, people with chronic pain may need to restrict their intake of some foods since they can worsen inflammation. Dietary factors such as high-processed foods, sugary snacks, and excessive red meat consumption have been linked to inflammation.

To ensure a comprehensive approach to pain management that goes beyond medicine alone, healthcare experts frequently collaborate with patients to develop individualized food programs that take into account their unique pain situation.

To sum up, knowing how food and medicine interact is essential to maximizing treatment results and guaranteeing patient safety. A key component of comprehensive healthcare is the incorporation of dietary considerations into medical care, whether that means modifying diets for efficient pain management or taking into account how specific meals affect the metabolism and absorption of drugs. Patients should be informed about these interactions by their healthcare professionals so they can make decisions that will improve the efficacy of their treatment regimens.

CHAPTER EIGHT

EXERCISE AND RECOVERY

THE VALUE OF MODERATE EXERCISE

Rehabilitation and physical activity go hand in hand; both are essential to preserving and regaining function, health, and general well-being. The value of moderate exercise is one of this domain's core ideas. In the case of patients recovering from surgeries, injuries, or long-term medical disorders, gentle exercise is an essential part of the rehabilitation process. It entails low-impact exercises and motions designed to increase circulation, flexibility, and mobility without putting the body under unnecessary stress.

The importance of mild exercise comes from its capacity to accelerate recovery, stop new injuries, and improve general physical function. Walking, swimming, and light stretching are examples of exercises that not only aid in the healing of particular muscles and joints but also improve the psychological state of patients undergoing rehabilitation. Gentle exercises are accessible to a wide range of people across different age groups and fitness levels because they can be customized to meet the unique needs and limits of each individual.

DIETARY ASSISTANCE FOR RECOVERY

Another crucial component of the rehabilitation process is nutritional support. The body needs proper nourishment to promote tissue regeneration, aid in recuperation, and restore energy resources. A well-balanced diet is crucial for patients undergoing rehabilitation to guarantee that the vital vitamins, minerals, and nutrients needed for healing and recovery are available. Consuming enough protein is especially crucial since it promotes muscle growth and regeneration, which aids in the restoration of strength and function.

Apart from protein, micronutrients including vitamins and minerals are essential for the general well-being of patients undergoing rehabilitation.

These nutrients support the preservation of bone density, aid in the healing process, and strengthen the immune system. Working together, nutritionists and medical practitioners can create customized meal programs that meet the unique requirements and objectives of patients undergoing rehabilitation.

INCREASING STURDINESS AND ADAPTABILITY

To improve mobility and lower the chance of recurrent injuries, developing strength and flexibility is a crucial part of the rehabilitation process. Exercises that build muscle strength and enhance joint stability are essential for people healing from ailments like fractures or operations. Stretching exercises and other flexibility exercises increase the range of motion and help reduce stiffness, which leads to increased mobility.

Exercise regimens that are specifically tailored to a person's current physical condition, restrictions, and rehabilitation objectives should be created with an emphasis on strength and flexibility building.

To progressively develop joint flexibility, muscular strength, and total functional capability, focused stretching exercises and progressive resistance training can be used. Physical therapists or other licensed healthcare providers oversee the safe and efficient execution of these workouts.

The fields of physical activity and rehabilitation heavily rely on the ideas of improving strength and flexibility, providing nutritional assistance, and engaging in gentle exercise. Together, these elements provide a comprehensive recovery that takes into account a person's dietary and physical needs. Healthcare providers can maximize the likelihood of a successful recovery and long-term well-being for patients undergoing rehabilitation by implementing these ideas into their programs.

CHAPTER NINE

TRANSITIONING GRADUALLY TO A REGULAR DIET

TRACKING DEVELOPMENTS WITH MEDICAL PROVIDERS

A gradual shift to a regular diet is important, and part of that process is tracking progress with healthcare specialists. When evaluating a person's health, medical specialists are essential in making sure that the reintroduction of food fits that person's unique requirements and medical conditions. Frequent evaluations and discussions with doctors, dietitians, or nutritionists facilitate the monitoring of advancements, detection of any obstacles, and modification of the food regimen as needed.

REINTRODUCING FOODS GRADUALLY

Comprehensive care requires cooperation with healthcare providers during the shift to a regular diet. Maintaining regular contact with medical professionals enables food plan modifications depending on individual reactions and evolving health situations. A comprehensive approach to health is ensured by monitoring progress through discussions about mental and emotional well-being in addition to physical assessments.

One of the most important strategies for going from a restricted or specialized diet to a typical one is to gradually reintroduce foods. This method entails gradually reintroducing items that have been excluded to gauge the body's reaction. People can keep an eye out for any negative responses or sensitivities by introducing one kind of food at a time. With the use of this technique, trigger foods may be identified with greater accuracy, and the normal diet can be modified to suit personal tastes and tolerances.

Foods must be gradually reintroduced with a methodical and careful approach. Starting with foods that are easily absorbed and do not cause gastrointestinal distress, the variety is progressively increased as the person's tolerance is evaluated. This method makes it possible to create a regular diet that is more individualized and customized by helping to discover particular items that may be uncomfortable or produce negative reactions.

LONG-TERM NUTRITIONAL GUIDELINES

Following the gradual change, long-term dietary guidelines are essential to maintaining a healthy lifestyle. These suggestions are frequently based on a person's medical history, particular dietary requirements, and general health objectives. Guidelines for keeping a balanced diet, controlling portion sizes, and including a range of nutrient-dense foods can all be found in long-term dietary regimens. The focus on a sustainable and well-rounded diet guarantees people's well-being even after the initial phase of change.

The goal of long-term dietary advice is to maintain general health and stop diet-related problems from happening again.

These suggestions could be in the form of instructions for sustaining a varied and nutrient-rich diet, adding frequent exercise, and forming sustainable lifestyle practices. The goal is to establish a pleasurable, well-balanced eating schedule that respects both personal tastes and cultural norms.

The methodical reintroduction of foods, long-term dietary guidelines, and progress monitoring with healthcare providers are all important components of the gradual shift to a regular diet. This collaborative and systematic approach provides a smooth transition, aids in recognizing individual needs, and sets the foundation for a sustainable and healthy lifestyle. Regular communication and adjustments with healthcare professionals contribute to the ongoing well-being of individuals as they embrace a diverse and balanced regular diet.

www.ingramcontent.com/pod-product-compliance
Lightning Source LLC
Chambersburg PA
CBHW060816260726
48660CB00002B/982